Table of Contents

Anyway, have you heard of the 'Banting Diet' previously? In the event that not, you might be surprised to know that this particular diet plan comprises of food things that are Low in Carbohydrates and High in Fat! Yes, High in Fat! The Banting Diet is more commonly known as Low Carb High Fat (LCHF) Diet as well. In typical diet plans, the very notice of the word 'Fat' is thought about a no-no, whereas if you follow Banting Diet Plan, you will constantly intake high fat food sources. Although it sounds very extraordinary, almost opposing, to other popular diet plans that we experience every day, it is widely accepted among circles of people who are conscious about their physique and fitness. What's more, that is so in light of the fact that there is considerable evidence that such a diet works wonders and is more viable than the traditional, low fat eating routine plans.Now, you may be pondering of the hypothesis behind this diet plan! What is Banting? Where does 'Banting' come from? The word 'Banting' became famous as a result of an undertaker, a royal undertaker who had proudly taken over the job of his forefathers. Like many of his kindred Londoners, Banting was a fat man for reasons that he shared with other obese people; the intake of heaps of sweet and sugary food sources. After retiring from his prestigious job in 1862, he was very depressed on the grounds that of his increasing obesity and grave health conditions that included hearing and site issues.

He could not get up the stairs on his own and was suffering from a ton of wellbeing issues.He himself is detailed to have written in his diary that fat is man's "insidious creeping enemy". At the time, the awareness about heftiness being linked with new unsafe diseases was also rising. Therefore, determined Banting left no stone unturned to get in shape and get rid of his corpulent body. After unlimited endeavors and practices such as strolling, riding on a horseback, avoiding fatty foods, he got in contact with a doctor, William Harvey, who recommended a novel plan for Banting. Although Banting showed much resistance to his diet plan that included food varieties rich in fats, the doctor kept on insisting him to eat butter, milk, potatoes, bread and so on Banting followed his specialist's diet for all three suppers in a day consistently and so, bore amazing results. The outcome of Banting Diet was just unbelievable.Now, he could go up the steps on his own. His defected hearing and sight improved a lot. Hence, he found a solution to his Big Fat Problem. Afterward, he distributed a short flyer telling his story, which spread throughout Europe and so, by 1866 quite a bit of Europe was caught by Banting-lunacy!

History of banting diet

It has been billed as a world-initial, an unique health culmination and heavenly assembling of low-carb, high-fat (LCHF, aka Banting) sustenance scientists, doctors and analysts from around the globe under one rooftop at the Cape Town International Conference Centre from February 19 to 22. Speakers at the Old Mutual Health Convention will look at the science, the ongoing controversy, and what works and doesn't work for sustenance in health and healing. In other words, how best food can be medication, and medication can be food, according to the injunction by the ancient Greek sage, Hippocrates.The high-fat summit's host is Prof Tim Noakes, a South African clinical doctor and internationally renowned scientist who has created intense interest and just as extraordinary criticism and visceral attack for changing his mind on the role of carbs in the eating regimen four years prior, in favour of low-carb, high-fat eating. Here, Noakes he gives the history behind the global LCHF movement, background to his own journey, the origins of the Cape Town meeting, background to the speakers, and what he trusts the Summit will achieve: 'a statement that will be heard around the world'. The beginnings of the Old Mutual Health Convention can be followed to William Banting and his monograph Letter on

Corpulence first published in London in 1862. His was the first description of the effective inversion of (resistant) stoutness with a reduced dietary sugar intake.Predictably William Banting's book was not eagerly embraced by the clinical calling in Britain. Attempts to have his idea distributed in the leading medical diary, the Lancet, were rebuffed. How possibly could a commoner know that which the medical calling did not? In time professional pressure forced the true creator of Banting's low carbohydrate eating plan, Dr

William Harvey, to write a book in which he stated that the benefits of his diet were not due to an increased fat content however were the outcome of its high protein composition.Banting deviated, stating that the key to his effective weight loss had been the higher fat content of Harvey's original diet. It was left to German physician and Professor of Medicine at Gottingen University, Dr Wilhelm Ebstein, to publish the authoritative description of the original low carbohydrate high fat diet in his 1884 monograph, Corpulence and its treatment on physiological standards. There he wrote:"This property of fat to produce satiety more rapidly, to diminish the craving for food and abate the feeling of thirst, facilitates to an extraordinary degree the presentation of the modified diet... The authorization to appreciate certain things, consistently of course in moderation, as for instance salmon, pate de foie gras and such like delights reconciles the overweight gourmet to his other penances (which) consist in the exclusion of carbohydrates. Sugar, desserts of all kinds, potatoes in every form I forbid genuinely. "The quantity of bread is restricted at most to 3 to 3 1/2 oz. a day, and of vegetables I allow asparagus, spinach, the various kinds of cabbage and especially the leguminous, whose esteem as conveyers of albumen (protein)... is known to few. Of meats I exclude none, and the fat in the flesh I do not wish to be stayed away from, however on the contrary looked for after. I grant bacon fat, fat roast pork and lamb, kidney fat, and when no other fat is at hand I recommend marrow to be added to the soup. I permit the sauces also as the vegetables to be made juicy, as did Hippocrates, only for his sesam-oil I substitute butter.

The Banting Diet works by increasing fats and decreasing carbs – a process that should encourage the body to consume fat. While following the plan, individuals are allowed to devour around 1900 calories a day. A long haul solution rather than a short-term fix, it aims to reduce hunger by making it easier for the individual to eat fewer calories. By cutting out most grains, processed foods and sugars, it's claimed the Banting Diet also helps balance blood sugar levels.According to Professor Tim Noakes in the book The Banting Pocket Guide, the diet can be tailored to suit different needs. He says: 'The level of carbohydrate intake can be adapted to the individual, and for those who are concerned about the consumption of too much soaked fat, there is the option of using monounsaturated fats like extra-virgin olive oil. 'The Banting diet was first recommended to William Banting in 1862 by Dr. William Harvey as a weight loss diet. William Banting's success with the diet led him to compose a booklet that popularized the low carb procedure for weight reduction, to the extent that the word "banting" became the name of the strategy, as well as a verb. Recently, Tim Noakes, a South African scientist and teacher, brought the method back into the spotlight after trying the Banting diet himself and composing the book "Real Meal Revolution." His take on the diet is alluded to as Banting 2.0.

The unique Banting diet included four daily dinners, which mainly contained protein and restricted carbs — 1 ounce (30 grams) of dry bread in each meal and 2–3 ounces (60–90 grams) of fruit as a snack. It limited bread, beans, spread, milk, sugar, beer, and potatoes. In any case, Tim Noakes' approach is somewhat unique. Banting 2.0 divides the process into four phases — observation, restoration, transformation, and protection — and offers multiple food lists and organized dinner plans to simplify the low carb approach. It actually limits carbs somewhat, and its macronutrient creation resembles the keto diet with under 5–10% of your every day calories coming from carbs, 65–90% from fat, and 10–35% from protein. Still, both versions of the diet guarantee outrageous weight loss, higher energy levels, improved sleep quality, reduced feelings of hunger, and increased feelings of by and large well-being.

Besides weight loss and great food, Banting has other benefits. It claims to reverse Type 2 diabetes and assists in controlling blood sugar in patients with Type 1 diabetes. It also claims to improve symptoms of IBS, Acne, Skin Irritations, PCOS and Heartburn. By simply cutting carbs and adjusting your diet by increasing the nutritional value of your foods, you can make a real change to your health and wellness. There are some concerns about adopting a

Banting approach to food though. Heart and Stroke Foundation South Africa, the Association for Dietetics in South Africa and other health groups are warning the public about possible health risks associated with the Banting diet. While they are still conducting their studies, these associations are concerned about increased risks of heart disease, strokes, cancers and diabetes that could possibly come with a LCHF diet. While they concede that certain fats are beneficial to heart health, they cannot endorse a LCHF diet plan until their research has concluded and they can unequivocally determine whether it is as healthy as Professor Noakes claims. Banting is also not recommended for everyone. It is not safe for women who are breastfeeding as it affects the amount of milk you produce and could lead to ketoacidosis – a life-threatening condition in which the body runs out of insulin. You should also consult your doctor before adopting Banting if you are on any diabetes or blood pressure medication, as the diet and the medication could result in dangerous complications.

We recommend consulting with your doctor before adopting the Banting lifestyle, even if you are not breastfeeding or on medication. It is dangerous to start a diet or make lifestyle changes without a thorough examination of your overall health so if you are interested in Banting, call your doctor first. Medical expenses to tend to stack up when you first adopt a lifestyle change – you will need to consult with your doctor in order to establish whether your diet is having any adverse effects on your cholesterol, blood pressure, blood sugar or other biological systems. Affinity Health offers affordable medical insurance options which could cover the costs of doctors visits and hospital stays. Adopting a diet can be challenging but Banting does make it much easier to shed the pounds and improve overall health and wellness while keeping the hunger pangs at bay. With banters in over 150 countries and some truly astounding results, Banting has become the first choice for many dieters around the world – and with the scrumptious meal options, we can't blame them.

The purpose of the diet is to keep the body slim and healthy. The diet's aims are limiting carbs, and eating more healthy fat and protein. Doing this also helps to reduce the risk of developing high blood pressure and hypertension, diabetes, and other chronic illnesses. It is a simple road to rejuvenate your health and stimulate weight loss. What the diet involves is the consumption of only "real food": food that is in its natural state and is unprocessed. In order

to follow the diet, you will need to do the following:

Avoid sugar and artificial sweeteners

Cut out burgers, pizzas, fries, and other fast food

Eat healthy fat like olive oil, nuts, and avocados

Avoid toxic oil like canola and sunflower

Decrease your intake of carbs

Consume a moderate amount of protein from eggs, fish, and meat

Eat more green vegetables like broccoli, cauliflower, and beans

The good, and the not-so-good of banting. When it comes to a new fad diet or trend, we're not easily convinced – nope, not at all. But with a lot of chatter in the health world surrounding the rather old, but new Banting Diet, which claims fat is not the enemy and weight loss is easy, we admittedly perked up and wanted to know more. So what is all the fuss about? Well firstly, it's not to be confused with the Paleo Diet though they both do encourage eating "real" foods rather than processed and refined food-like substances. The name is derived from Mr William Banting himself, a London undertaker who in 1861 was prescribed a weight loss plan that consisted of low carbohydrate, high fat food (LCHF). But it wasn't until Dr Robert Atkins appeared with his famous Atkins Diet in 1972, did eating fat start to rise in popularity. Since then the diet has been dusted off and re-worked, and now with banting-friendly restaurants popping up all over South Africa and social media goers like Banting Babe giving it a try, it seems everyone is on-board the banting train.

The Banting Rules

There are no tedious recipes or complex calculations with this one – the principles are simple: eat foods that are high in fat, low in carbohydrates and are medium in protein. Only eat when you're hungry and stop when satisfied. Sounds easy enough, right? Well, before you sign along the dotted lines there are a few big no's to be mindful about. There is no sugar, no grains (of any kind), no fruit or very little, and definitely no snacking allowed. You can also say goodbye to that afternoon beer or cider, too.

But what you can do is, embrace the love for foods like avocados, coconut oil, eggs, fatty fish (these are the good fats). And be sure to stock up on proteins like salmon, lentils and chicken. Dairy foods such as yoghurt, milk and cheese are okay (phewf!).

How to follow the Banting diet

The Banting diet is divided into four phases that are meant to ease the transition into a LCHF way of life.

While you may follow the diet on your own, there's an online course available for those who want to dive into it with a structured and personalized Banting meal plan.

The course offers a step-by-step guide, recipes, optional daily support from a coach, and weekly mindset workshops to help manage temptations and make the transition smoother.

Phase 1: Observation

During this 1-week phase, you're supposed to follow your current diet without making any modifications. It encourages you to track and journal everything you eat to figure out how you respond to food.

Phase 2: Restoration

The restoration phase is meant to restore your gut health and get you used to the Banting way of eating.This phase may last 2–12 weeks, depending on your weight loss goal. Overall, you should follow it for 1 week for every 11 pounds (5 kg) of weight you want to lose. During this time, you'll be introduced to a series of food lists. You're meant to eliminate all foods from the Red and Light Red lists and instead rely on those on the Green and Orange lists. One plus is that there's no calorie counting or portion control in this phase.

Phase 3: Transformation

The transformation phase introduces you to the original Banting diet. It takes your newly developed eating habits and cuts your carb intake to achieve ketosis, which is meant to get you into a rapid fat-burning mode. To make this possible, the method encourages you to stick to foods on the Green list, while adding those on the Orange list to the no-go foods — along with the Red lists mentioned before. This third phase lasts as long as it takes you to reach your desired weight, and you should track your meals for a couple of days every two weeks. Additionally, the phase includes "lifestyle hacks," such as intermittent fasting, exercise tips, and sleep and meditation to avoid reaching a weight loss plateau. The transformation phase is supposed to improve mental clarity, sleep, acne, and skin irritations, as well as even eradicate joint pain.

Phase 4: Preservation

This final phase, which is supposed to last indefinitely, starts once you've reached your desired weight. It's meant to help you maintain your new weight in the long run. This is a more flexible phase, as you'll be able to reintroduce foods that are not allowed in the previous phase. The goal is to determine which ones you can safely eat without gaining weight.

Again, there's no food tracking during this phase, and you may follow the food lists as follows:

Green: no limitations

Orange: eat in moderation

Light Red: hardly ever or on special occasions

Red: never

Gray: it's up to you

You can always return to the previous phase if you feel like you have lost control of your weight

The Banting diet provides multiple food lists to eat and avoid.

Green list

This list includes foods that you may eat without restriction.

Fruits and vegetables: leafy green vegetables, artichoke hearts, aubergine, asparagus, bean and Brussels sprouts, broccoli, green beans, cabbage, cauliflower, celery, chard, courgettes, cucumber, endive, fennel, garlic, germ squash, kale, leeks, lemon and lime, lettuce, mange tout, mushrooms, olives, onions, okra, palm hearts, peppers, radicchio, radishes, rhubarb, rocket, shallots, spinach, spring onions, snap peas, tomatoes, and turnips

Meat, fish, and poultry: all meat, poultry, fish, seafood, offal, and naturally cured meats (i.e., pancetta, salami, parma ham, bacon, jerky, coppa (capocollo), and biltong), eggs, homemade bone broth, and cheeses, such as

Brie, Camembert, Gorgonzola, Roquefort, mozzarella, feta, ricotta, Cheddar, Gouda, Emmental, Parmesan, and pecorino

Drinks: caffeine-free herbal teas, flavored waters, and plain water

Condiments: all kinds of vinegar and fermented soy sauce or tamari

Fermented foods: coconut yogurt and kefir, kefir butter and cheese, kimchi, milk kefir, naturally fermented pickles, and sauerkraut

Fats: any rendered animal fat, avocado, butter, ghee, cream, coconut oil, fruit and nut oils, mayonnaise, and seeds

Orange list

According to the method, foods on the Orange list offer multiple health benefits but may hinder your weight loss journey if consumed without restriction. Thus, foods on this list are meant to be enjoyed in moderation.

Nuts: all raw nuts and sugar-free nut butters

Dairy: milk and milk substitutes, cottage and cream cheese, full fat yogurt, and sour cream

Fruits: apples, apricots, bananas, blueberries, blackberries, cherries, clementines, fresh figs, gooseberries, granadilla, grapes, guava, jackfruit, kiwi, kumquats, litchis, loquats, mangoes, nectarines, orange, papaya, pears, peaches, persimmon, pineapple, plantain, plums, pomegranates, quinces, raspberries, starfruit, strawberries, tangerines, tamarind pulp, and watermelon

Drinks: caffeinated tea and coffee

Legumes and pulses: all legumes, alfalfa, beans, chickpeas, and lentils

Fermented foods: water kefir and kombucha

Fruits and vegetables: beetroot, butternut squash, baby corn, carrots, calabash, cassava, celeriac, corn, edamame, golden beets, Hubbard squash, jicama, parsnips,

peas, potatoes, pumpkins,
rutabagas, spaghetti squash, and
sweet potatoes

Light Red list

You should hardly ever consume
foods on this list.

Smoothies and vegetable juices:
fruit and yogurt smoothies without
frozen yogurt or ice cream, as well
as vegetable juices without added
fruit juice

Treats and chocolate: dark chocolate (80% and above), dried fruit, honey, and pure maple syrup

Gluten-free grains: amaranth, arrowroot, buckwheat, bran, gluten-free pasta, millet, oats, popcorn, quinoa, rice, sorghum, quinoa, tapioca, and teff

Flours: almond, coconut, corn, chickpea, pea, and rice flours, polenta, and maize meal

Red list

This is probably the most important list, as it includes the foods you should never eat.

General foods: fast food, foods with added sugar, chips, and sugary condiments, such as ketchup, dressings, and marinades

Sweets: all confectionery and non-dark chocolates, artificial sweeteners, agave, canned fruit, coconut sugar, cordials, fructose, glucose, jam, malt, rice malt syrup, sugar, and golden syrup

Gluten: barley, bulgur, couscous, durum, einkorn, farina, graham flour, Khorasan wheat (kamut), matzo, orzo, rye, semolina, spelt, triticale, wheat, and wheat germ

Grain-based products: all commercial breaded or battered foods, breakfast cereals, and all crackers

Drinks: energy drinks, soft drinks, commercial juices, commercial iced teas, flavored milks, and milkshakes

Dairy-related foods: coffee creamers, commercial cheese spreads, condensed milk, ice cream, and commercial frozen yogurt

Fats: butter spreads, canola oil, corn oil, cottonseed oil, margarine and shortening, rice bran oil, and sunflower and safflower oil

Processed meats: highly processed sausages and meats cured with sugar

Gray list

The Gray list contains foods that fit the Banting diet but would slow your progress, so they're left to your discretion.

Treats: Banting baked goods and sugar-free ice cream

Sweeteners: xylitol, erythritol, isomalt, stevia powder, and sucralose

Drinks: all alcoholic beverages, protein shakes, and supplements

Vegetarian proteins: naturally fermented tofu, pea protein, and processed soy

Banting Diet Shopping List

The results are going to be tremendous as long as you stick to the diet. Be diligent and be honest to yourself at the beginning, and listen and respond to your body.

Like many diets, this diet can be hard work. But, get the grasp of it and it will be smooth sailing with happy and healthy results.

Banting Diet Grocery List

Green List

Protein

All meat

Eggs

Seafood

Vegetables

All green leafy vegetables

Artichokes

Broccoli

Cabbages

Cauliflower

Cucumbers

Celery

Garlic

Lettuce

Mushrooms

Radishes

Tomatoes

Drinks

Caffeine free herbal drinks

Flavored water

Sparkling water

Orange List

Fruit

Apples

Bananas

Cherries

Grapes

Oranges

Papaya

Peaches

Pumpkins

Mangos

Vegetables

Baby corn

Beetroot

Carrots

Corn on the cob

Nuts

Peas

Dairy

Cottage cheese

Cream cheese

Feta cheese

Milk

Milk substitutes (coconut, almond, soy etc.)

Mozzarella

Ricotta

Drinks

Coffee

Tea

10 commandments of the Banting Diet

All you need to know before you start this change to a healthy lifestyle;

Consume animal fat

This is the focal point of the Banting Diet. This challenges the way we think because we have always been taught that fat makes us fat. The truth is that sugars and refined carbohydrates causes insulin spikes which tells your body to store energy as fat.

Consume as much vegetables as possible

 Vegetables are known as the 'bulk food' to all Banters. Green veggies are the go-to-vegetables and all banters know that eating a variety of these veggies is the best for the body.

Snacking is a big No-No unless its Banting Friendly

Snacking is a form of cheating especially when on the first week of Banting. Try not to snack unless its Banting-friendly. The solution to beating down those hunger pangs is to increase the amount of animal fat intake as fat acts as a natural appetite suppressant.

Never lie to yourself

Consuming high carbohydrate foods that are professed usually hide in foods such as peanuts, baked beans and legumes. Refer to the "Banting Diet red list; foods that should not be consumed as a Banter" to make sure you stay within the guidelines.

Never over eat and never under eat

Beginner Banters have a habit of either eating too much or too little. Just because you are confined to a low carb diet it doesn't mean you can eat as much fat as you like. At the end of the day if you eat more calories than you burn you will still put on weight. On the other hand don't under eat while being on the Banting Diet. Fat contain fewer calories compared to carbohydrates so you will probably need to eat more than you expect. If you become extremely hungry during the Banting diet chances are you are either under eating or you have not been eating enough fat. The great thing about this diet is fat is a lot more filling than carbohydrates so you shouldn't feel much hunger at all if done properly.

Try not to consume too much protein

The Banting diet is a high fat, low carb diet and NOT a high protein diet. The main point of the Banting Diet is to cut out the carbohydrates from your diet and replace it with more fat. Don't focus on increasing your protein intake. You will naturally get enough protein with all the vegetables and meat you will eat.

Always read Food Labels

Always be on the lookout when it comes to ready made meals or processed foods. These foods almost always contain carbohydrates. Stay away from foods that claim they are low in fat. These foods may be low in fat but the fats have been replaced with sugars to compensate for the loss of flavor. "Low Fat Meals" are nothing but a sly marketing tactic.

Avoid consuming too many fruits and nuts.

Fruits contain natural fructose which is "natures sugar". On the

Banting diet ANY sugar should be limited, if not avoided completely.

Nuts can be found on the Banting Diets green list however like any food they should still be eaten in moderation. People tend to over eat nuts because they make the perfect snack to carry around all day.

Control the amount of dairy you consume

Dairy does contain carbohydrates, and yes, it can be good for the body however is should be strictly controlled and moderated. Dairy does contain small amounts of carbs therefore its not a free for all. If you are lactose intolerant avoid dairy all together.

Remain strong

A lot of people tend to give up early while being on the Banting Diet. The first 10 days in this diet venture are always the most difficult because your body is still in the process of getting rid of those nasty carb cravings. Stick with it, after 10 days when the carb cravings disappears you'll start seeing drastic changes, not just with your weight but also your over all mood.

7 Day Banting Diet Meal Plan

Monday

Breakfast

2 eggs (fried)

Few rashers of bacon or pork sausage

Tomato

Lunch

Large salad with steak or chicken and cottage cheese

Snack

Apple slices with almond butter

Dinner

Pork with steamed spinach and pumpkin and a small tub of Greek yoghurt

Tuesday

Breakfast

Omelette with bacon, cheese, rocket and tomato

Lunch

Sautéed vegetables

Snack

Small can of tuna

Dinner

Greek salad with olive oil

Broccoli or cauliflower with cream cheese

Steak

Wednesday

Breakfast

Eggs and bacon

Coconut milk smoothie

Lunch

Green leafy salad

Chicken breast

Snack

Yoghurt

Dinner

Roast chicken

Pumpkin with butter

Baby marrow with cheese
sprinkled on top

Thursday

Breakfast

Scrambled eggs in butter

Few rashers bacon

Mushrooms, onions, tomato and pepper friend in bacon fat

Lunch

Biltong salad with full cream yoghurt

Snack

Hard boiled eggs

Dinner

Fish and some prawns

Spinach and pumpkin and a Greek
salad

Friday

Breakfast

Banana pancakes

Coconut smoothie

Lunch

Vegetable soup

Snack

Biltong

Dinner

Beef or chicken
Stir fried vegetables in olive oil

Saturday

Breakfast

Yoghurt and berries smoothie

Lunch

Egg and sweet potato hash browns

Snack

Mixed raw nuts

Dinner

Hake friend in butter and lemon juice

Spinach with butter and garlic

Grilled pumpkin

Sunday

Breakfast

Eggs

Bacon

Mushrooms fried in olive oil

Lunch

¼ chicken

Cucumber and tomato slices

Snack

Avocado

Dinner

Steak

Roasted butternut

Spinach

While there's no research on the Banting diet itself, there's plenty of scientific evidence supporting the LCHF approach for weight loss. When restricting carbs, the body is stimulated to maximize fat oxidation to meet energy demands. This means that LCHF diets rely primarily on fats to produce energy. Research suggests that there may be two different mechanisms behind the LCHF diet's success — increased feelings of fullness and a specific metabolic advantage. Studies show people on LCHF diets given unrestricted access to foods don't necessarily consume more calories than people on low fat, high carb (LFHC) diets because they tend to perceive less hunger, and thus, reduce their overall food intake. Additionally, LCHF diets usually lead to a higher protein intake, which also promotes feelings of fullness, and fewer cases of rebound hypoglycemia or low blood sugar levels, a common cause of hunger in those following high carb diets. Regarding the alleged metabolic advantage, scientists attribute it to either an increased thermogenic effect from the protein intake, a higher protein turnover for gluconeogenesis, or loss of energy through the excretion of ketones in sweat or urine. The thermogenic effect of foods is the energy needed to digest, absorb, and dispose of its nutrients, while gluconeogenesis is the production of glucose from fats or proteins.

Also, by eliminating foods on both Red lists, you're more likely to lose weight faster, since processed and sugary foods are associated with excess weight.

Finally, the lifestyle hacks mentioned above, such as intermittent fasting, can also contribute to weight loss, as it has been shown to increase metabolism and help burn more fat .

The Banting Diet is one of the many low-carb, high-fat (LCHF) diets to go mainstream.

To help you know if LCHF diets are for you, here are some of the reported health and lifestyle benefits they may offer:

Long-Term Weight Loss Compared to HCLF Diets:

Studies suggest that LCHF diets may be more effective at achieving long-term weight loss goals than high-carb, low-fat (HCLF) diets.

Reduced Metabolic Risk:

Several studies show that LCHF diets may help reduce the risk of cardiovascular disease (CVD), diabetes and obesity.

Improved Weight Loss vs. HCLF Diets:

Studies show that LCHF diets may slightly improve weight loss efforts compared to HCLF diets when both include reduced caloric intake.

Help Reduce Acne:

In some cases, acne breakouts can be triggered by processed and refined carbohydrates. LCHF diets may aid in reducing these types of skin outbreaks.

Additional benefits

Following a LCHF diet like the Banting diet may lead to other potential health benefits.

Improved metabolic markers

LCHF diets may help reduce risk factors for both type 2 diabetes and heart disease.

Scientific evidence shows that they may reduce fasting insulin and blood sugar levels and improve insulin sensitivity, which is why LCHF diets are gaining popularity as potential first-line treatments for type 2 diabetes.

They also seem to decrease triglyceride and high blood pressure levels, increase HDL (good) cholesterol, and reverse nonalcoholic fatty liver disease.

For example, in one 12-week study in 26 people with excess weight, those following a LCHF diet improved their glucose, insulin resistance, triglyceride, HDL (good) cholesterol, and HbA1c levels, compared with those in the HCLF group.

The HbA1c test — or glycated hemoglobin test — measures your average blood sugar levels over the past 3 months, and it's used as an evaluation tool for blood sugar control in people with diabetes.

Focuses on wholesome foods

By restricting processed and sugary foods, the diet almost automatically leads to a higher intake of wholesome, more nutritious foods.

High intakes of processed foods are associated with increased oxidative stress and inflammation, leading to the development of non-communicable chronic diseases (NCD) like cancer and heart disease and thus increasing the risk of mortality.

On the contrary, healthy eating patterns that focus on increasing fruit and vegetable intake seem to decrease the risk, as their nutrients help reduce oxidative stress and inflammation.

Potential downsides

While the Banting diet offers numerous health benefits, its potential downsides cannot be ignored.

Highly restrictive

Aside from eliminating processed and sugary foods, the Banting diet's food lists also restrict grains and limit fruits, legumes, dairy, and nuts.

Evidence shows that consumption of those food groups may be beneficial for the prevention of type 2 diabetes, heart disease, and certain types of cancer.

Additionally, by restricting legumes, dairy, and nuts, and classifying tofu as a "gray area food," the diet makes it difficult for vegans and vegetarians to follow the plan.

Finally, the restrictive nature of the diet can make long-term maintenance difficult, which could end up hindering its effectiveness.

However, some may find that the support from online communities or the course's coaches and webinars is all they need to keep them going.

Long-term evidence is lacking

While the benefits of a LCHF eating patterin like the Banting diet seem promising, there's not enough human evidence to support its safety in the long run.

Some human and animal studies suggest potential adverse long-term effects of LCHF diets on LDL (bad) cholesterol levels and blood vessel elasticity, which may be detrimental to heart health.

However, more research is needed to understand how low carb diets affect heart health over longer time periods.

Therefore, some believe that the potential downsides of following this type of diet in the long term outweigh its potential benefits.

Ingredients

12 deboned chicken thighs, cut into 3 and seasoned well with salt and pepper

4 tbsp butter

1 onion, finely chopped

1 leek, finely chopped

1 stalk of celery, finely chopped

2 cloves garlic, crushed

1 cup dry white wine

1 cup chicken stock

1 cup cream

1 tsp dried Italian herbs

1 tbsp dijon mustard

for the pasta

600 g courgettes, sliced into ribbons with a potato peeler

3 tbsp butter

Directions

Melt the butter in a large pan and brown the chicken until it is golden. Remove from the pan and set aside.

Turn the heat down to medium and add the onion, leek, celery and garlic to the pan and gently fry until they are soft.

Add the white wine and let it simmer and reduce by half.

Add the chicken stock and let it simmer for 5 minutes.

Finally add the cream, dried herbs and mustard and let the sauce simmer for a few minutes.

Add the chicken to the sauce and cook for 5 minutes.

To make the noodles: Melt the butter in a large frying pan and toss the courgette through. Keep frying until the courgettes are warmed through. This should be quite quick.

Serve the chicken poured over the courgettes.

Ingredients

6 large eggs boiled; cooled; peeled; and cut in half

1 avocado mashed

3 slices bacon cooked and crumbled

1 tbsp Jalapeno pepper finely diced

1 tsp red onion finely diced

2 tbsp tomato chopped

1 tbsp lime juice

1 tbsp cilantro (coriander) chopped

1 dash salt and black pepper to taste

1 pinch cayenne pepper to taste

1 dash chilli powder for garnish

Directions

Scoop the yolks out of the egg halves, mash them, mix with the avocado, bacon, jalapeno, onion, tomato, lime juice and cilantro and season with salt, pepper and cayenne.

Place a tablespoon of the mixture
back into the holes left by the yolks
in the eggs and serve garnished
with extra bacon and a pinch of
chili powder.

Ingredients

1 Cauliflower broken up into of florets (approx 5 cups)

2 Cups of grated cheddar cheese (preferably organic from grass fed cows)

1 Cup of coconut milk

2 Tbsp coconut flour

1 Egg (free range)

½ Cup homemade broth

Salt & pepper for taste

2 Cloves of garlic (optional)

Directions

Pre-heat your oven to 180°C
(350°F)

Steam the cauliflower florets, add
salt & place in a greased baking
dish

Warm the coconut milk & add the
broth whilst keeping stirring

Add the coconut flour to the
mixture & allow it to bubble

Remove it from the heat & add in
the beaten egg

As the mixture begins to thicken
pour it over the cauliflower florets
in the baking dish

Add the grated cheese evenly over
the cauliflower

Place the dish into the pre-heated oven & bake for 30 to 40 minutes

Finally grill the dish for a few minutes to get a nice golden colour on top

Banting Cabbage and Mince

Ingredients

3 tbsp Butter, unsalted

500 gm Beef, ground

1 medium Yellow onion (chopped)

1 large pepper(s) Red bell pepper ((seeded and chopped))

3 clove(s) Garlic (chopped)

1 can(s) (28oz) Diced tomatoes, canned (or fresh tomatoes)

1/2 tsp Paprika (smoked)

1/2 tsp Oregano, dried

1 pinch Salt and pepper (to taste)

1 small head Green cabbage (cored and chopped)

2 cup, shredded Cheddar cheese

Directions

Saute beef, onion and sweet pepper in butter over medium/high in a large pan with high sides or a dutch oven. Cook until beef is browned and onions are translucent.

Add garlic and saute 1 more minute.

Stir in tomatoes, spices, salt and pepper. Top with cabbage. Cover and cook 15-20 minutes or until cabbage is tender.

Top with cheese, cover until melted then serve.

Ingredients

2 Tbsp Coconut Oil

1 large Onion chopped

1 Tbsp Crushed Garlic

500 Beef Mince (preferably 80/20 i.e. 20% fat - if lean, add more coconut oil or butter)

1 Tin Chopped Tomatoes

2 Tbsp Dried Origanum (or other herbs of choice)

2 Tbsp Dried Sweet Basil (or other herbs of choice)

Salt and pepper to taste

Directions

Heat a medium sized pot up.

Add Coconut Oil and heat then sauté onions until translucent.

Add garlic and sauté.

Add mince and fry until cooked and well broken up.

Add herbs and stir.

Add tomato and cook on low for about 20 minutes. If you need to add more liquid, add a little water.

Easy Low-Carb Cauliflower Fried Rice

Ingredients

2 tablespoons butter, ghee, coconut oil, or olive oil

12 ounces riced cauliflower fresh or frozen

1/4 cup carrot finely diced (optional)

1 ounce green onion (about 2 large or 4 small) sliced, with white and green parts separated

2 cloves garlic crushed

1 large egg beaten

2 tablespoons gluten-free soy sauce or Tamari (more or less to taste)

1 teaspoon toasted sesame oil

Directions

In a large heavy skillet or wok, melt butter or oil of choice over medium-high heat.

Add carrots and riced cauliflower. Cook, stirring occasionally, until vegetables begin to soften--about 5 minutes.

Stir in the white part of the green onions. Cook until vegetables are almost tender--about 2-3 minutes more. Add the garlic and cook for 1 minute.

Pour in the egg and stir it together with the vegetables. Cook, stirring the mixture frequently, until the egg is scrambled. This takes about 1-2 minutes.

Stir in the soy sauce, green part of green onions, and the sesame oil. Taste and adjust seasoning.

EASY MOZZARELLA CHICKEN

Ingredients

4 5-ounce (150 gram) boneless skinless chicken breasts

1 tablespoon Italian seasoning

1 teaspoon paprika

1/2 teaspoon onion powder

Salt and pepper, to season

1 tablespoon olive oil

1 onion, chopped

4 cloves garlic, minced

1 fire roasted pepper, (fire roasted capsicum), chopped

15- ounces 425 grams crushed tomatoes, OR tomato puree (Passata)

2 tablespoons tomato paste, garlic and herb flavoured if possible

Pinch crushed red pepper flakes OPTIONAL

3/4 cup shredded mozzarella

1 tablespoon freshly chopped parsley, to garnish

Directions

Arrange oven shelf to the middle of the oven. Preheat broiler (or grill in Australia) on medium heat.

Season chicken with 2 teaspoons of Italian seasoning, paprika, onion powder, salt and pepper.

Heat oil in a pan or skillet over medium heat. Cook chicken on both sides until browned and cooked through (about 8 minutes each side). Transfer to a plate; set aside.

Cook the onion in the same pan until transparent (about 3-4 minutes) scraping any browned bits form the bottom of the pan, then add in the garlic and cook until fragrant (about 1 minute). Add the fire roasted pepper (or capsicum), crushed tomatoes, tomato paste, crushed red pepper flakes (if including) and remaining Italian seasoning. Give it a good stir to mix well.

Bring to a simmer and allow the sauce to thicken while stirring occasionally (about 4 minutes).

Arrange the chicken in the sauce and top each breast with 2-3 tablespoons of mozzarella cheese per breast. Transfer to the oven to broil for 1-2 minutes, or until the cheese in browned and bubbling.

Garnish with parsley and serve.

Ingredients

Banting pizza base:

- 1 cauliflower
- 1 egg
- 1 cup (250ml) grated mozzarella
- 1 tbsp (15ml) psyllium husk
- ¼ cup (60ml) almond or coconut flour
- Salt and milled pepper

Bacon, mushroom and spinach topping:

- 4 rashers streaky bacon, chopped

- 1 cup, (about 125g) button mushrooms, sliced

- 1 clove garlic

- Pinch dried chilli flakes

- ¼ cup (60ml) grated Edam cheese

- Salt and milled pepper

- Handful baby spinach

Directions

Banting pizza base:

Cut the cauliflower into smaller florets and lightly steam. Pulse in a food processor to create crumbs. Take care not to

over-blend or you will end up with purée. Alternatively, you can steam ready-crumbed cauliflower.

Should the cauliflower retain any water, place it in a clean dishcloth and twist to remove all the liquid.

Mix the cauliflower with the remaining ingredients.

Line a baking tray with baking paper or a silicon sheet.

Place 'dough' onto the baking sheet and press out into desired shape.

Bake in a preheated oven at 200ºC for 15 minutes, or until golden.

Bacon, mushroom and spinach topping:

Add a splash of oil to the pan.

Fry bacon until crispy.

Add mushrooms, and cook for about 5 minutes. Add garlic and chilli. Cook until mushrooms are soft.

Scatter cheese over pizza base, top with bacon mixture and season.

Bake, until cheese is bubbling.

Top with a handful of spinach, and serve.

Low-Carb Creamed Spinach

Ingredients

600 g fresh spinach (1.3 lb)

2 tbsp butter or ghee (28 g/ 1 oz)

1/3 cup mascarpone cheese (80 g/ 2.8 oz)

salt and pepper, to taste

1/4 tsp nutmeg

1/3 cup grated Parmesan or other Italian hard cheese (30 g/ 1.1 oz)

Directions

Bring a large pot of water to a boil. Blanch the spinach for 30 to 60 seconds. Immediately plunge the spinach into a bowl filled with ice water.

Drain well, pat dry, and set aside.

Place the butter and mascarpone in a saucepan, and add the blanched spinach and combine.

Add salt, pepper to taste and nutmeg. Gently heat until it begins to simmer.

Then mix in the Parmesan.

Serve topped with more grated Parmesan. Optionally, you can place under the broiler for 2 to 3 minutes, until crisp and lightly golden. Serve immediately or let it cool down and store in the fridge for up to 3 days.

INGREDIENTS

Butter

6 x Eggs

1 Cup Marscapone Cheese

Packet of Bacon

1 Onion Chopped

1 Packet of washed baby spinach

Directions

Preheat oven to 180°C.

Grease a muffin pan using butter.

Rinse and chop your favourite bits
(I used onions, bacon & spinach)

In frying pan, sauté your favourite
bits until cooked and slightly
browned. Once cooked, set aside.

In a mixing bowl, whisk eggs on
high speed with salt & pepper, add
the marscapone cheese and blend
well.

Fill bottom of muffin pan about 2cm with your sautéed bits and pouring egg mixture over this until muffin pan just under full.

Place in oven and cook for 20 minutes or until golden brown.

Allow to cool

Once cooled, slide a flat butter knife around the edges to loosen the sides and remove from the pan.

Enjoy!

Ingredients

Braai Meat Mix(chicken wings, Vors & chuck)

2 Tablespoon Cajun spices(carbwise)

1 teaspoon salt

1 teaspoon pepper

2 Tablespoon Braai salt(carbwise)

Directions

Seasons all your meat with your Spices and let it rest for 20 minutes.

Make sure your fire is not hot too much so that your meat does not burn, avoid turning the meat to much. Enjoy

Ingredients

2 tablespoons coconut flour

2 tablespoons golden flax meal

3/4 cup water

pinch of salt

1 large egg beaten

2 teaspoons butter or ghee

1 tablespoon heavy cream or coconut milk

1 tablespoon Low carb brown
sugar or your favorite sweetener

Directions

Measure the first four ingredients
into a small pot over medium heat
and stir. When it begins to simmer,
turn it down to medium-low and
whisk until it begins to thicken.

Remove the coconut flour porridge
from heat and add the beaten egg,
a half at a time, while whisking
continuously. Place back on the

heat and continue to whisk until the porridge thickens.

Remove from the heat and continue to whisk for about 30 seconds before adding the butter, cream and sweetener.

Garnish with your favorite toppings. (4 grams net carbs)

INGREDIENTS

2 zucchini, thinly sliced lengthways

4 (about 255g each) beef scotch fillet or porterhouse steaks

1 tbs coarsely ground black pepper

1 tbs coarsely chopped thyme

2 tbs red wine vinegar

1/4 cup (60ml) avocado oil or olive oil

2 tsp wholegrain mustard

120g baby spinach leaves

330g jar whole roasted peppers (capsicum), drained, torn into strips

100g blue cheese, crumbled

Thyme sprigs, to serve

Directions

Heat a barbecue grill or chargrill on medium-high. Spray the zucchini slices with olive oil spray. Cook the zucchini slices on the grill for 1 min each side or until lightly charred. Transfer to a plate.

Spray the steaks with olive oil spray. Sprinkle with the pepper and chopped thyme. Season with salt. Cook steaks on grill for 2-3 mins each side for medium or until cooked to your liking. Transfer to a plate and cover with foil to keep warm. Rest for 5 mins. Thinly slice.

Meanwhile, whisk the vinegar, oil and mustard in a small jug. Season.

Place the zucchini, spinach, capsicum and blue cheese in a large bowl. Gently toss to combine.

Divide the salad and steaks evenly among serving plates. Drizzle the salad with the dressing and sprinkle the steaks with thyme sprigs to serve.

Seitan and broccoli stir-fry

INGREDIENTS

2 tablespoons Shaoxing wine

1 tablespoon light soy sauce

2 teaspoons caster sugar

2 teaspoons cornflour

60ml (1/4 cup) peanut oil

250g seitan, sliced (see notes)

2 teaspoons finely grated fresh ginger

2 garlic cloves, finely chopped

1/2 teaspoon chilli paste

200g broccoli, cut into florets

Sesame oil, to drizzle

Sliced green onions, to sprinkle

Steamed rice, to serve

Directions

Combine the Shaoxing, soy sauce, caster sugar, cornflour and 1 tablespoon of water in a small jug. Set aside

Heat the peanut oil in a wok over high heat. Cook the seiten in 3 batches for 2 minutes each batch, or until crisp. Transfer to a plate.

Drain all but 1 tablespoon of oil from the wok. Add the ginger, garlic and chilli paste and stir fry for 30 seconds or until aromatic. Add the broccoli and 2 tablespoons of water. Stir-fry for 3 minutes or until the broccoli is crisp and the water has evaporated.

Add the soy sauce mixture and seiten and stir fry for 1 minutes or until the sauce has thickened. Drizzle with sesame oil and sprinkle with green onion. Serve with rice.

Mexican zucchini slice

INGREDIENTS

5 eggs

3 egg whites

3 teaspoons Mexican spice mix

2 zucchini, grated

1 large carrot, grated

4 green shallots, thinly sliced

80g (1/2 cup) frozen peas, thawed

40g (1/4 cup) self-raising flour

1/2 cup chopped fresh coriander, plus extra leaves to serve

60g chedder cheese, coarsely grated

1 avocado, sliced

1 tomato, cut into wedges

Sriracha, to drizzle

Directions

Preheat the oven to 200C/180C fan forced. Grease a 26cm ovenproof frying pan with oil.

Whisk the eggs and egg whites in a large bowl until combined. Add spice mix and season well. Add zucchini, carrot, shallot and peas. Add flour, coriander and half the cheese. Stir until combined.

Pour mixture into prepared pan and sprinkle with the remaining cheese. Bake for 20-25 minutes or until golden and cooked through.

Top with avocado, tomato and extra coriander. Drizzle with sriracha

Ingredients:

1/2 cup flaxseed

1/2 cup sunflower seeds

1 1/2 cups almond flour

2 tablespoons psyllium husk powder

1/2 cup buttermilk

1/2 cup sour cream

1/2 cup Greek yogurt

6 eggs

2 tablespoons baking powder

1 tablespoon salt

2 tablespoons finely chopped nuts

Directions

Put the flaxseed and sunflower in a food processor. Process until very fine.

Combine the flaxseed mixture with the almond flour.

Chop and add the psyllium husks.

In a separate bowl, combine the buttermilk, sour cream, Greek yogurt and eggs.

Slowly add the buttermilk mixture to the flaxseed mixture. Stir well with a wooden spoon after each addition.

Add the salt and baking powder.

Flour and grease a loaf pan. Pour the mixture into it.

Bake at 350 degrees for 50 minutes.

Top with chopped nuts. Return pan to oven and continue to bake about five minutes until a wooden stick inserted into the center comes out clean.

Banting Spice Bread

Conclusions

The Banting diet is a type of low carb, high fat (LCHF) diet that mostly restricts boring, handled, and sweet food varieties, rather promoting the consumption of wholesome ones to lose weight rapidly. Despite the fact that there's no logical evidence on the eating regimen itself, studies on LCHF counts calories suggest that they may enhance metabolic markers for heart disease and diabetes. All things considered, the diet is highly restrictive, and there's not enough proof on the long-term effects of LCHF diets in people. Therefore, maintaining a intake of wholesome food varieties and reducing your intake of prepared ones while shifting to a moderate-carb diet may be a more sustainable yet proficient weight misfortune approach.